MEN'S SELF HAIRCUT

A step by step practical guide with pictorial illustrations for men

Nedu Anukam

Copyright © 2019 Nedu Anukam

All rights reserved.

ISBN: 9781705404157

DEDICATION

Dedicated to my family, friends and all men wishing to acquire new skills for a happier life.

CONTENTS

ACKNOWLEDGMENTS

Putting this work together was supported and made possible by the concerted efforts of my friends, family members and graphic designers who contributed immensely through valuable inputs, designs and proof-reading. I must say thank you in a special way.

OVERVIEW

Giving yourself a haircut is a valuable skill that saves both time and money. On average, it costs between $15 to $30 or more per week to have a haircut in a barbing salon. That means in a year, you would have spent between $720 and $1,440 on haircut. This is okay for those who can afford it and have the time, however, if you haven't got the time or wish to be more prudent in your spending, it is worthwhile doing it yourself and that is the sole purpose of this book.. Doing it yourself may not necessarily be for financial reasons but also to keep yourself busy at leisure times with something meaningful. The skills you acquire by learning to cut your own hair is not only useful to you but also useful to your children as you can give them a clean haircut without taking them to the salon. As your children grow older, you can transfer your skills to them by training them to give themselves a haircut. It is a once and for all skill that comes with immense benefits in terms of knowing that you or your children don't have to travel to the salon to spend money on haircut, giving you the freedom to care for yourself in the comfort of your home at any time.

I give myself and family members a perfect and stylish haircut in the comfort of my home and I have been doing it perfectly for over a decade as a hobby. Although I can afford to go to the salon and pay to have a haircut, but I feel more satisfied and comfortable doing it myself. It takes patience and regular practice to gain mastery of the process.

The various stages involved in achieving a clean and decent haircut are explained in simple and comprehensive terms with pictorial illustrations used as much as possible to illustrate the processes and to advance your understanding. Learning to give yourself a haircut is more effective practically than reading this book. Thus, the more you practice the better your improvement and results. The most important thing is motivation, patience and practice.

Benefits of Self Haircut

- ✓ **It is a valuable skill**
- ✓ **It saves you a lot of money**
- ✓ **It gives you more freedom and flexibility**
- ✓ **It can be done in the comfort of your home**

STAGE ONE

Instruments

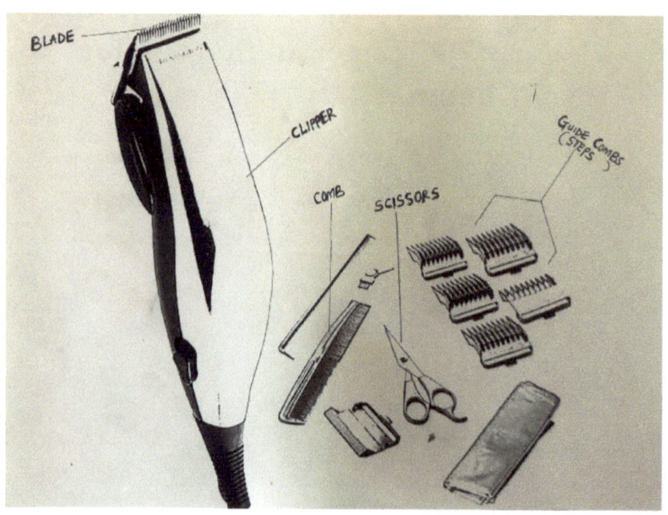

Giving yourself a haircut is different from someone else doing for you, hence using the right instruments is necessary to achieve a good result. Without the right instruments, it is difficult to do it by yourself and you will most likely end up with a bad result. Fortunately, the instruments are cheap and available at your local supermarkets.

Three-Way Mirror: A three-way mirror is

essential and considered a modern way of facilitating a better self-haircut. A three-way mirror is designed to enable you to see all parts of your head/hair without holding the mirror. It may be purchased online or at your local supermarket

Two Mirrors: Using two separate mirrors is considered an old fashion, however, it is still very effective and preferred by most people. For your comfort, the two mirrors should be big and small. The big mirror (40 to 50 inches in size) or just big enough to see your entire back and top of your head clearly should be placed on the wall behind you. The small hand mirror should be held closely in front of you in your left hand. You can see every part of your head/hair from the small hand mirror by moving your head in different directions

Hairbrush or Comb: A hairbrush may be suitable if your hairs are short or not too grown. A hair comb may be used if your hairs are long or well grown. Prior to starting your haircut, it is advisable to brush or comb your hair as many times as possible to loosen and soften them. It is also advisable to keep your hairs are dry as possible.

Hair Clipper: This is locally available in most supermarkets. For better results and safety, it is advisable to buy an original and durable hair clipper. Most hair clippers are already fitted with a sharp or self-sharpening blade. The blade can be adjusted forward and backward to achieve different levels of sharpness/ different low-level haircut.

Forward adjustment = Less sharp blade, less skin-level haircut

Backward adjustment = sharp blade, skin-level haircut.

Note that the blade adjustment result may vary depending on the thickness or softness of your hair, so a gentle application is required. Hair clippers are sold with four guide combs of different sizes that are attached to the shaver head. **The guide combs come in 3 different sizes designated step 1, 2, 3, 4 or more.** Step 1 is the smallest and normally used to achieve the lowest haircut, followed by step 2, 3 or more, which are used for medium and long hairs.

A Pair of Scissors: This may not be necessary if your hairs are not long. I personally do not use scissors because I have no long hairs to trim down. However, if your hairs are long, scissors may be used to trimming or levelling.

Aftershave Cream: It is advisable to have this cream handy before having a haircut to prevent bumps from developing on your scalp. This may be available at chemist /pharmaceutical stores near you.

Instrument Hygiene

It is necessary to practice and maintain a high standard of instrument hygiene before and after haircut to minimise or eliminate the risk of infection. Before starting your haircut, ensure that your clipper blades, scissors and all skin piercing instruments are sterilized. Affordable and portable sterilization equipment may be purchased online from reliable stores. After your haircut, keep your clipper and scissors clean by brushing off hair particles around them.

Direction of Hair Growth

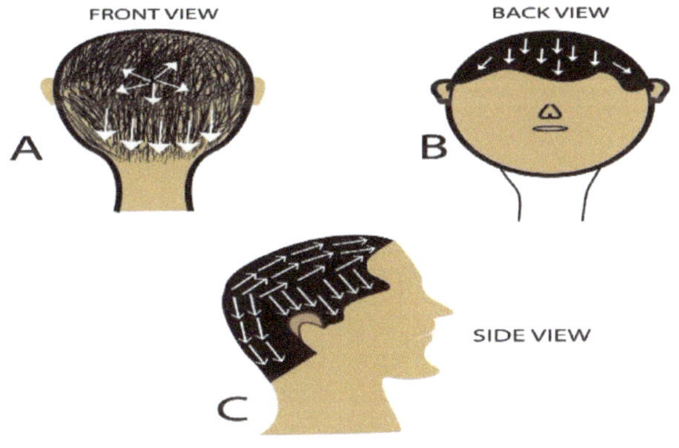

The above diagram illustrates the directions of hair growth. Generally, hairs begin in a spiral form from the top central part of the head (**diag. A**) and grow in different specific directions as illustrated above. Hairs on the top front part of the head (**diag. B**) grow mainly forward towards the face, while hairs on the top back of the head (**diag. A**) grow mainly downwards towards the back of the neck. Hairs on the sides of the head (**diag. C**) grow downwards towards the ears (C). For diagram B, it is best to cut in the direction of hair growth, from the top central part of the head moving towards the face. Hairs on both sides of the head and back (**diag. A & C**) can be cut from any direction to suit your intended style.

STAGE TWO

Starting Your Haircut

Begin by brushing/combing your hair to soften and straighten. **A three-way mirror** is essential and required for flexibility and a clear view of all areas of your head/hair. As stated earlier, three-way mirror is considered a new fashion in self haircutting because you do not necessarily need to hold a mirror in your hands to see your hair. However, the old method of using two mirrors is still very effective and preferred by most people. In this method, a bigger mirror is placed behind you, while **a smaller mirror is held in your left hand** and **a hair clipper in your right**

hand.

Three-way mirror

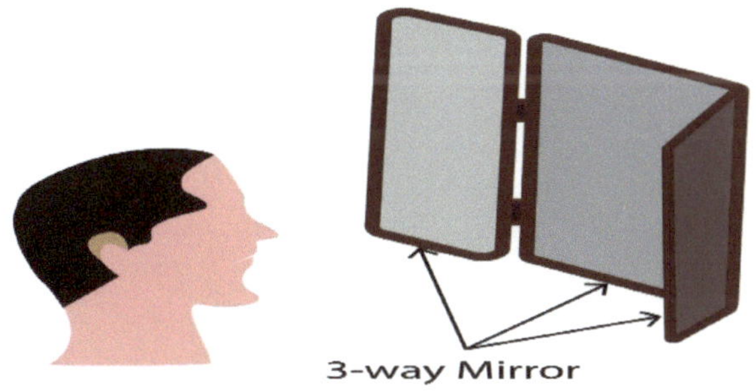

Old method with two mirrors

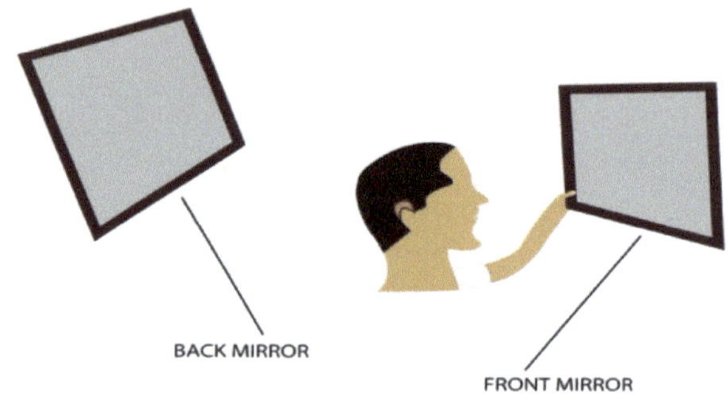

U-Shaped Line Formation

The first step is to form a u-shaped line with the clipper blade adjusted backwards to achieve a reasonable sharpness. The guide combs/steps are not required at this stage. **The arrows (diag. A and C) indicate the direction of the blade.** Cut gently to skin level, starting from the neck region at the back or **from the mid part of the ear as a landmark** on each side of the head, moving upwards until a u-shaped is formed.

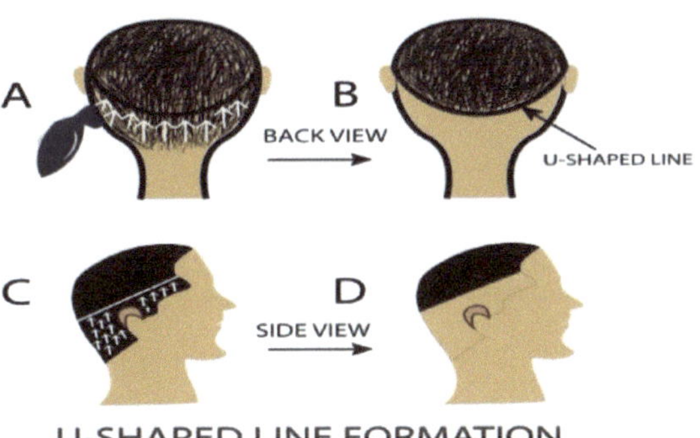

U-SHAPED LINE FORMATION

The line on both sides of the head should stop just **behind the top part of the ears** and joins in a straight regular pattern with the line at the back to form a u-shape as shown in diagrams B and D. You may follow this starting procedure regardless of the length of your hairs and your goal. The next step involves getting rid of the line without damaging the u-shape.

Line Fading

When the u-shaped line is faded, it faints and disappears but still retains the image of a u-shape and forms 3 layers as shown in diagram D. The arrows (diag. A) indicate the direction of the blade for fading.

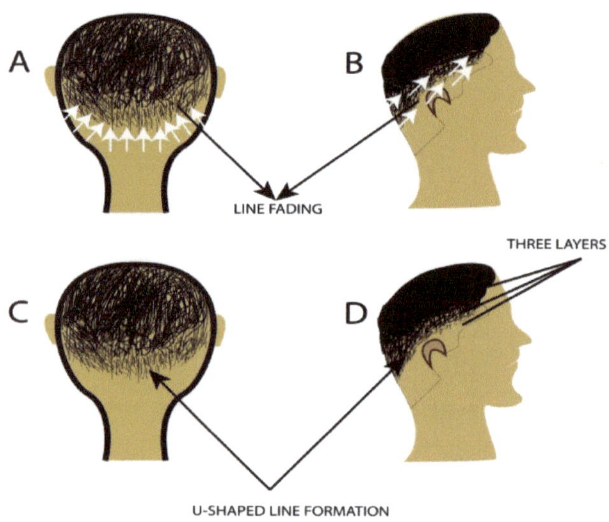

Greater care is required during fading to avoid damaging the entire process. Using the arrows as a guide, begin by gently, slowly and softly fading vertically without pressing the blade hard on the line. The same result can be achieved by fading horizontally. The blade should be gently placed directly on the line either vertically or horizontally (see arrows in diag. A and B). If done correctly, three layers will be formed as shown in diagram D. The final step involves levelling the first layer (1.)

STAGE THREE

Levelling the First Layer

Once the 3 layers have been formed, the first later which is the topmost and longest part of the hair may be levelled to give a flat and even surface, with no hairs longer than the others. To achieve this, the guide comb steps 2, 3 and may be 4 may be used depending on how low you want to go. For longer hairs, steps 3 and 4 may be suitable.

THREE LAYERS

The direction of the arrows in diagram (E) indicates the direction of your clipper blade so this should be used as a guide. Cut gently and superficially from back to the front without digging the blade dip into the hairs until your desired level is reached. The lower you cut, the smaller the guide combs/steps needed for better result, and the longer your hair, the bigger the guide comb/steps required. A pair of scissors may be used at this stage to level the top part of your hair, but this is optional if you attach the right guide comb/steps to the blade and maintain the same adjustment for the entire part of your hair being cut.

Trimming

This is the final step of your haircut. It is easier to trim your hair than giving yourself a full haircut, so it should be an easier part of the process.

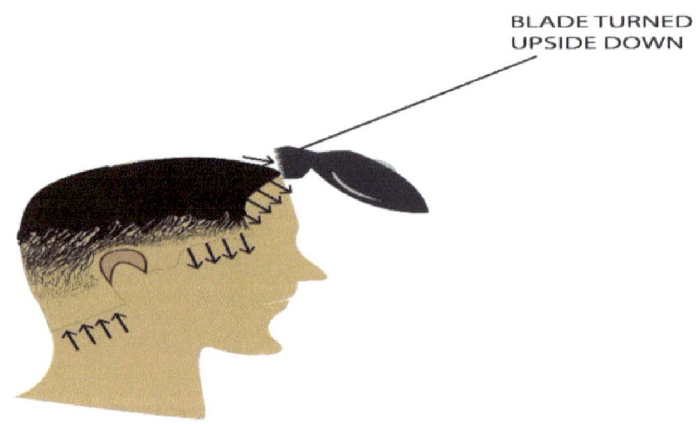

Begin by turning the clipper/blade upside down as shown above and trim towards the direction of the arrows in the diagram for the front and side hairs trimming. Notice that the arrows at the back of the head and those at the top and side parts of the head are facing different directions. Follow the direction of the arrows on each area when trimming. The clipper / blade should be turned back to its normal position when trimming the back

Front part of the hair = Outward trimming

Side part of your = Outward trimming

Back part of your hair = Inward trimming

It is a lot easier to have the clipper/blade facing the normal way (not turned upside down) when trimming the back of your hair. It may be turned upside down when someone else is doing the haircut. After trimming, remember to apply your aftershave cream, lubricate your clipper blade with the right clipper oil and secure.

CONCLUSION

The basic concept and procedures illustrated in this book will enable you to give yourself a stylish three-layered, two-layered or one-layered haircut. The more you practice, the more confident, comfortable and faster you become at giving yourself a haircut. Do not be discouraged when you make mistakes since your hairs will always grow back. If you make a serious mistake trying to achieve a three-layered or two-layered hair style, the best option I would suggest is to go on a single-layered style and wait for your hairs to grow back in a week or two, and then try again.

I hope you enjoyed reading and learned something new from this book. It is now time to put everything to practice.

I wish you the best of luck!

About the Author

Nedu Anukam, is well experienced in self-haircutting. He's been a self-barber for more than a decade, giving himself a haircut as well as helping friends and family members acquire the skill to keep themselves busy with something meaningful at leisure, and save money by not having to visit the barbing salon regularly. The author believes that having the skill to cut your own hair adds personal and economic value to your life and makes you more content and happier.